I0439757

Essential Oils for Beginners: Aromatherapy Recipes for Weight Loss & Well-being

Contents

Introduction

I want to thank you and congratulate you for downloading the book, *"Essential Oils for Beginners: Aromatherapy Recipes for Weight Loss & Well-being"*.

This book contains proven steps and strategies on how to use various essential oils to help you achieve your weight loss goals, reduce stress and solve minor skin and hair problems.

If you use essential oils, you can be sure that the products you use for your well-being are completely natural. Further, since essential oils are very concentrated, you only need to use a small amount every time so you can save money in the long run.

Thanks again for downloading this book, I hope you enjoy it!

Chapter 1 – What Are Essential Oils?

Before we discuss how essential oils can benefit your well-being, let us first discuss what they are. This is important because too many people mistake artificial fragrance oils for essential oils then experience unpleasant complications after using them.

Essential oils are hydrophobic, i.e. water-repelling or do not completely dissolve in water, substances distilled from various plant parts like leaves, flowers, stems, bark, roots, or the whole plant. Chemically speaking, they are not true oils because they do not contain fatty acids unlike olive and coconut oils. They are only called oils because they resemble oil in the sense that they are hydro-phobic. However, they are not necessarily oily or greasy. In fact, some essential oils can resemble water in appearance because they are colorless and not viscous. On the other hand, some essential oils can feel oily when applied on the skin and have a thick consistency.

They are called *essential* oils because they contain the essence of the plant. If you look at the chemical composition of any plant, you will see that it contains water, cellulose or the plant fibers which give it structure, and its essence or what makes it the plant that it is. You can consider the essence to be the concentrated nutrients of the plant.

To make essential oil, you must first boil the plant to extract its essence then further boil the water to distill the essential oil. This is a difficult process which is why most people opt to buy their essential oils rather than make them even if they are fortunate to have a garden which supplies them with various plants and herbs. Sometimes people will simply boil the plant and use this 'tea' for various purposes, or they will infuse oils with the plant to extract some of its goodness. While these methods can be effective, the amount of plant essence in the 'tea' or infused oil is very minimal. Hence, it might take a while before any improvement is seen. In contrast, since essential oils are concentrated, it can take as little as a few days to see improvement.

Each plant can only give a small drop of essence. For example, to make 10 ml. of lavender essential oil, you need about 150 grams of lavender flowers. This is why essential oils tend to be on the expensive side especially if they are organic. However, since you only use a small amount every time, you will actually be able to save money in the long run. You only need to use at most 3 drops at a time depending on what you are using the essential oils for. A 10 ml. bottle which generally costs around $20 can last about a year or longer.

Chapter 2 – Some Precautions When Using Essential Oils

Before you go out and buy essential oils, you have to take note of some important considerations:

First, it is very important to understand that just because something is natural it doesn't mean it cannot do any harm. People too often forget that most poisons and irritating substances are 100% natural like snake venom, poison ivy and poison oak. So what is the advantage of using natural products?

When you use natural products, you can be sure that you are not contributing to the destruction of the environment. Natural products break down naturally to be reused by nature in some other way. This is not to say that all artificially created substances are non-biodegradable, rather you can be 100% sure that you are not contributing to more non-biodegradable waste than necessary unlike when you use non-natural products.

You might ask, 'Is that all?' The truth is, yes, that is the gist of it. Anyone who says that natural products are safer is only trying to make you buy their product. Natural products are not necessarily safer because they can still result in irritations especially if they are used incorrectly, and people can still be allergic to them. However, do not think that using natural products is not worth it just because you only get one advantage, and it isn't even a direct advantage to you. Nowadays, nobody can afford to not care about the environment. By using natural products, you can help to save the environment even in a small way.

Second, you have to ensure that you are buying *true* essential oils rather than artificial fragrance oils. The latter are oils which have been artificially scented. They are used for cheap soaps and other bath products, and sometimes for oil burners and scented candles. To the untrained nose, artificial lavender fragrance oil can smell like true lavender essential oil, so it is possible to be duped into buying them.

This is very dangerous because if you are going to use this oil on your skin or if you intend to ingest it, you might hurt yourself. The oil base used for these artificial fragrances might be extremely irritating to the skin and it can contain impurities which may poison you if you ingest it.

Unfortunately for most essential oil newbies, too many stores label their bottles of artificial fragrance oils as essential oils. Sometimes they do this so they will be able to sell their products for a higher price, but sometimes the sellers themselves do not know what exactly they are selling because the term 'essential oil' is now commonly used to refer to both true essential oil and artificial fragrance oils. It is also possible that they buy their oils from disreputable sources.

You should be wary of stores selling cheap essential oils because they are likely artificial fragrance oils.

Recall that it takes a lot of plants to make a small amount of oil. If so, then anyone who sells a 10 ml. bottle of essential oil for only $5 will not make any profit. Since this doesn't make any sense, it is best to assume that the product is not true essential oil.

On the other hand, it is possible that the product is on sale. There is nothing wrong with taking advantage of sales, but take note that essential oils should be treated like medicine or food. They do not last forever. Either they will lose their effectivity or the scent will change. Citrus oils like lemon and grapefruit usually only last for a year while oils made from wood or bark like sandalwood can last up to 5 years. It is possible that the bottles of essential oil are on sale because they are about to expire. It is all right to buy them if you use them up quickly, but if not you might only end up throwing your money down the drain.

The only way to know for sure that you are getting true essential oil is to chemically test it. Experienced noses can usually detect a slight difference between true oils and artificial ones, but even they cannot be 100% sure. Since most people don't have chemistry laboratories at home, the best way to ensure that you are getting true essential oil is to buy from reputable sources.

The label should tell you where the plants used are grown, when the oil was made and when it will expire. Reputable brands cost more but if you will not buy food, medicines and beauty products from disreputable sources, then it makes sense to do the same when buying essential oils.

Third, depending on your purposes, you can buy pure or diluted essential oils, but it is still better to buy pure oils then dilute them yourself. Essential oils can be diluted with water, alcohol or oil. Bottles of diluted essential oil will cost less than pure oils, but they have their disadvantages. First, they cannot be used in a variety of ways. For example, pure lemon essential oil can be used to flavor food, to beautify the skin and even to polish furniture; but if it is mixed with a *non-food grade* olive oil, you can no longer use it to flavor food. However, if you only use your essential oils in limited ways, then you might find it all right to buy them diluted.

Another disadvantage of using diluted essential oil is you cannot tailor the concentration for your purposes. For example, a 10% tea tree oil solution mixed with vitamin E oil can be good for minor acne, but serious acne is still best treated with 100% or pure tea tree oil. If you suffer from large pimples and buy the diluted solution because you think this will save you money, you might as well throw that money away because 10% is not enough for your situation. Even if it turns out that the 100% solution is too harsh for you and you only need 50%, you can dilute the essential oil yourself, thus it will not be wasted.

Sometimes disreputable stores will sell diluted essential oil as 100% pure oil. They can easily fool newbies because they dilute the essential oil with distilled water or neutral smelling oil like grape seed oil. The only way to make sure you have pure essential oil is through chemical analysis.

Some people say you can use the 'paper test' to check for purity. This is done by placing a drop of essential oil on a paper towel then allowing it to dry. If an oily mark remains, the essential oil is not pure but has been diluted with oil. This test only works if the essential oil was diluted with oil, but it will not work if it was diluted with water. Also, some of the more viscous essential oils like sandalwood might leave an oily mark. Again, to avoid problems in the first place, it is best to buy from reputable sources.

Fourth, if you tend to be allergic to many things, it is best to start with only a small amount of essential oil. Once you are sure that the oil gives you no adverse reactions, you can increase the amount you normally use. We will discuss how to do this in the succeeding chapters. However, if you suffer from many skin and food allergies, it is best to stay away from essential oils.

Fifth, some essential oils have limited use. For example, tea tree oil can be applied on the skin but must never be ingested. Some, like wintergreen, must not be used on a long-term basis because this results in poisoning. Some must not be used for aromatherapy like camphor. Pregnant women should be especially careful since there are essential oils which are known abortives like sage. Also, even if an adult can safely use an essential oil, this is not necessarily true for children and pets.

The safest essential oil for all-around use is lavender oil; but experts still disagree on whether it is actually safe for pregnant women. To be on the safe side, avoid all essential oils during pregnancy except those which can be safely used for aromatherapy, but only for this particular purpose.

In this book, we will mention only the essential oils which are relatively safe to use. At any rate, the more dangerous essential oils are usually not easily available in stores. As a newbie, it is best to stick to the more common essential oils which have been tested as safe for most people.

Sixth, essential oils should be treated like food or medication. They usually come in opaque bottles but it is still better to keep them in a cool, dark place to help preserve them. It is not necessary to keep them in the refrigerator unless you live in a very hot and humid climate. If you choose to dilute or mix your oils with other substances, keep the solution in a sterilized, opaque glass bottle or jar. You can easily sterilize your containers by pouring boiling water over them then allowing them to dry.

This chapter is rather long but it is really necessary to mention all the precautions to avoid any problems. As was already mentioned, essential oils must be treated like medicine or food. They are not simply fragrant substances you can play with.

Chapter 3 – Essential Oils for Weight Loss

Before we discuss how to use essential oils for weight loss, you should understand that they can only *help* you lose weight. You cannot reasonably expect them to magically make your weight disappear overnight. When it comes to weight loss, regular exercise and a reduced calorie diet still play significant roles.

To use essential oils for weight loss, you have to ingest them. Doing this will slightly increase your metabolism to help you burn more calories. This does not mean you can eat a whole cake then simply allow essential oils to burn all the calories away. At most, you can expect essential oils to help you burn about 5% of your *reduced calorie diet*. For example, if you consume only 1500 calories daily to lose weight, essential oils will help you burn up to 75 calories even without exercise. The actual amount will depend on other factors but that is the maximum amount you can expect to burn.

If you think that 75 calories per day is too few, remind yourself that your body burned this amount even if you did not exercise. If you continue to use essential oils, you can burn up to 525 calories in a week and 2100 in a month even if you are only relaxing at home. Even if you are only able to burn

20 calories a day through the use of essential oils, that amount can still pile up.

Take note that you must already be on a reduced calorie diet. If you still consume too many calories daily, then even if essential oils help you burn about 5% of your total calories, the fact that you eat too much will still make you pack in the pounds.

The essential oils which can be used for weight loss include the following: grapefruit, peppermint, lemon, ginger, and cinnamon. They should be ingested either by adding them to your beverage of choice, or by adding them to your food.

If you choose to do this, make sure that your essential oil is *true* and *pure* essential oil, i.e. it is not artificial fragrance oil and it is not diluted. This is very important since you will be ingesting the essential oil. You do not want to poison yourself.

To use essential oils for weight loss, consume 1 to 2 drops of any of the above daily. Use only a maximum of 2 drops per day.

Here are some ideas:

- The above essential oils can be used to flavor water. Use 1 to 2 drops for every 8 ounces. Start with 1 drop during the first few days just to see how your body reacts. If you experience no adverse reactions like allergies or stomach cramps, add another drop. If you use 2 drops, you can either add both of them to 1 glass of water or you can add 1 drop each to 2 glasses of water to be consumed separately.

- Instead of water, you can use tea or fruit juice, but make sure the flavors go well together. Any of the above can be used with black, green or oolong tea, but they might not taste good with certain types of herbal teas. Grapefruit, peppermint, and lemon can be paired well with most fruit juices, but ginger and cinnamon can be tricky. Ginger is great with peach juice and cinnamon can be used for fruit smoothies blended with milk. If you prefer to drink coffee rather than tea, cinnamon is a great choice.

- If you take apple cider vinegar for its weight loss benefits (since it is able to boost your metabolism too), add 1 to 2 drops of any of the above essential oils to mask the sour flavor.

- You can choose to cook with your essential oils too. Use them to flavor salad dressings, sauces, marinades, porridge, desserts and baked goods. For example, if a recipe calls for lemon juice, add lemon essential oil instead. Just make sure that you use only a maximum of 2 drops for each serving. If the flavor is lacking, add lemon juice rather than more essential oil. You can also experiment with various flavors like adding some ginger essential oil to your soups for a fiery kick.

Chapter 4 – Aromatherapy for Wellbeing

Aromatherapy is the use of smells or aromas to cure certain ailments. Depending on the essential oil used, it can be used to cure nasal congestion, headache, dizziness, nausea, and many others. It can also be used to reduce stress and to stimulate the mind.

The question most people ask regarding aromatherapy is 'Is it ok to use artificial fragrance oils instead of true essential oil since it is only the scent you are after?'

The answer is 'It depends.'

In Chapter 2, we have discussed how it is better to buy true essential oils rather than artificial fragrance oils because you can use the former in a variety of ways and the scent is superior. However, if you only need the scent and promise to not use artificial fragrance oils for ingestion or on your skin, then you can use high quality fragrance oils (yes, there is such a thing) which smell almost like the real thing that only the most experienced nose can detect that they are artificial. It is even possible for the artificial fragrance to smell exactly like the real thing.

High quality artificial fragrance oils are actually used in the more expensive fragrances to enable companies to keep up with consumer demand. It is difficult to consistently produce large amounts of true essential oils because the available amount will always depend on the amount of plants harvested specifically for that purpose. In the end, the fragrance company might decide that it is more efficient for them to use high quality fragrance oils rather than to produce less of their product. Since the fragrance is only applied to small areas of the body, the chances of skin irritation occurring is less compared to skin care products scented with artificial fragrance oils.

However, here's the catch: high quality artificial fragrance oils can cost as much as true essential oils. Thus, you can make do with the former if you cannot find the latter *as long as you do not plan to use them on your skin like in the case of scented soaps and lotions.* As far as cheap fragrance oils are concerned, avoid them. They smell too artificial that you might end up with a worse headache.

The various ways you can use essential oils for aromatherapy include the following: heated in an oil burner or diffuser, inhaled directly, sprayed around the room and added to candles, soaps, lotions, massage oils or other body products. What is important here is you are able to smell the aroma.

The method you use will depend on what works for you and your personal preferences. For example, while direct inhalation will give you the most intense scent, this might be too much for some people. Oil burners, diffusers and candles are easy to use but they cannot be left alone because they are fire hazards. They must also be used properly. You should read the instructions before using them. Candles, especially the cheap ones, can sometimes not contain enough essential oil to have an effect. Room sprays and scented body products provide only a subtle scent which might not be very effective. You have to use trial and error to know what is best for you.

Meanwhile, here are the scents to look for depending on your concern:

- For general headaches choose peppermint, ginger, lavender, eucalyptus or roman chamomile. For headaches due to a cold, you can combine equal amounts of peppermint and eucalyptus. For stress headaches, use lavender and roman chamomile at a 2:1 ratio.
- For dizziness and nausea, sniff some roman chamomile.
- For nasal congestion, choose peppermint or eucalyptus. It is best to use an oil burner or diffuser for this ailment, or even to sniff the scent directly from the bottle. For maximum relief, combine equal amounts of both.
- To help manage stress, lavender is the best choice. You can also try sandalwood, rose and jasmine if you like very feminine scents. Lavender can also be combined with the other 3 in equal amounts. For a very feminine and sophisticated scent, combine rose, jasmine and sandalwood in a 2:2:1 ratio. However, this scent might not be effective for those who dislike feminine scents.

- To stimulate the mind and to help you concentrate, choose peppermint, lemon, orange, grapefruit or other citrus scents. If you feel stressed but at the same time must be able to concentrate, combine lavender and peppermint scents in equal amounts.

Chapter 5 – Essential Oils for Skin and Hair Care

Essential oils can also be used for a variety of skin and hair ailments. However, before we consider these, we must mention some precautions specific to the use of essential oils on the skin.

First, in Chapter 2, we already mentioned that those with a lot of skin and food allergies must avoid the use of essential oils. For those who do not suffer allergies, it is still possible to be allergic to something; only you don't know it yet. To be on the safe side, before using essential oils on your skin, do a skin test first.

To do a skin test, apply a very small drop of essential oil on a hidden part of your body like behind the ear or inside the elbow, then wait for 24 hours. If no irritation occurs, the essential oil is safe for you. If irritation occurs, wash the area with mild soap then repeat the process with a drop of diluted essential oil. Do this on a different part of your body. You can dilute the essential oil with distilled water or a little bit of body oil or lotion. Mix them in a small bowl or on the palm of your hand, then apply the solution with your finger. If irritation still occurs, then you should avoid that particular essential oil.

Second, most essential oils can be very irritating to the eyes. You should exercise great care when using oils on your face. However, rose and chamomile essential oils are generally safe to use around the eyes.

Here are some ways you can use essential oils for skin and hair problems:

- For acne, use pure tea tree oil or lavender oil directly on spots. If this is too harsh for you, dilute the essential oil with an equal amount of grape seed oil. This is the lightest available oil and is great for oily complexions. You can either mix them fresh every time you need to treat your skin, or you can mix them beforehand and keep the solution in a sterilized, opaque glass bottle. Make sure to shake your solution well before each use. For very oily skin or if you dislike the feel of oil on your face, you can also dilute the essential oil with distilled water or 50% ethyl or isopropyl alcohol. Take note though that alcohol can irritate sensitive skins.
- For fine lines and wrinkles, use lavender, rose, jasmine or sandalwood. You can either apply the pure oil directly on the affected parts, or you can combine it with a carrier oil to provide a more moisturizing effect.
- The term 'carrier oil' is used to refer to the oils used to dilute essential oils. Grape seed oil is best for oily skin. Dry skins can benefit from olive, coconut or argan oils, while normal skin can use jojoba or sweet almond

oil. Those with very oily complexions can use distilled water or alcohol as described above.

Take note that the effectivity of the essential oil is diminished if it is diluted.

- For dark under-eye circles, use rose or chamomile essential oil diluted with an equal amount of the carrier oil of your choice. Use your ring finger to dab this solution around your eyes every night. Do not use alcohol to dilute essential oils used for the eye area.
- For dark spots or acne marks, lemon essential oil is a good choice. Use it pure on the affected areas or dilute it with your choice of carrier oil. If you also suffer from fine lines and wrinkles, combine equal amounts of lemon essential oil with lavender. This will create a pleasantly feminine and uplifting scent.
- To help keep your complexion young-looking, add 20 drops of green tea essential oil to 10 ml. of vitamin E oil. Green tea and vitamin E are great antioxidants. Use this mixture as a moisturizer by spreading at least 3 drops all over your face. Use more if your complexion is dry or less if it is oily.
- For fungal infections like ringworm, use tea tree oil or lavender. It is best to use pure essential oil for this purpose; however, if your skin is very sensitive, you can dilute the essential oil with an equal amount of coconut

oil since this is also a known anti-fungal substance.

To ensure that the fungus is speedily killed, soak a gauze pad with the pure or diluted essential oil, then apply it on the affected part. Use a bandage to keep it in place.

- To prevent falling hair and to encourage hair growth, massage a solution of rosemary essential oil, aloe vera gel and olive oil on your scalp. Use 10 ml. each of aloe vera gel and olive oil then add 10 drops of rosemary essential oil. Shake the mixture well before using it. Do this at least once a week for best results.
- For dandruff or scalp psoriasis, mix 10 to 15 drops of tea tree, eucalyptus or lavender essential oil to 100 ml. of your usual shampoo. Shake this solution well before every use. You should feel a pleasant tingle on your scalp. Add more essential oil if necessary.
- For head lice, combine 20 to 30 drops of tea tree oil and 1 cup of coconut oil. The tea tree oil will kill the lice while the coconut oil will dissolve the cement attaching the nits to the hair shaft. Apply this mixture all over the hair and scalp then leave it for at least 1 hour. Afterwards, wash off the mixture. You might need to shampoo your hair 3 times to get everything off. This treatment should be repeated for at least 3 consecutive days or

until all traces of lice are gone. Meanwhile, bed sheets and clothes should be changed daily, and the hair should be combed with a fine-toothed comb to remove any remaining live lice.

Conclusion

In today's society we tend to live stressful lifestyles with little time for ourselves. Conditions such as stress can be a catalyst to many discomforts to our physical being. Aromatherapy in conjunction with essential oils can help relieve many common physical ailments as well as help us maintain emotional stability.

I do believe through experience, and the anecdotal proof offered to me by many of my friends and relatives that essential oils and aromatherapy can be most beneficial to your health.

I do not advocate that essential oils should replace conventional medicine, yet I do believe that they have a prominent role to play in maintaining general health and mental wellbeing. If you are in doubt it is always best to check with a qualified medical or aromatherapist before use.

I hope this book was able to help you with increasing your knowledge on how to use essential oils for various purposes.

The next step is to try the tips listed here to see what works for you.

Thank you again for downloading this book!

Bonus Content!

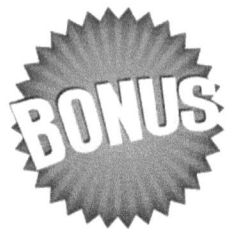

As a token of our appreciation <u>Grand Reveur Publications</u> would like to give you access to our exclusive bonus content (including free eBooks!).

<u>You're only a click away from receiving:</u>

Exclusive pre-release access to our latest eBooks

Free Grand Reveur eBooks during promotional periods

A method ANYONE can use to publish their own book and make passive income

https://ignorelimits.leadpages.net/grandreveur publications/

As this is a limited time offer it would be a shame to miss out, I recommend grabbing these bonuses before reading on.